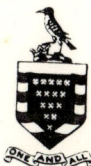

Talking to Your Doctor

CAROLYN FAULDER

Virago

London

Published in Great Britain by Virago Limited 1978
4th floor, 5 Wardour Street, London W1V 3HE

ISBN 0 86068 032 0

Printed and bound by Unwin Brothers Limited, The Gresham Press.
Old Woking, Surrey.

Contents

VIRAGO
is a feminist publishing company:

'It is only when women start to organize in large numbers that we become a political force, and begin to move towards the possibility of a truly democratic society in which every human being can be brave, responsible, thinking and diligent in the struggle to live at once freely and unselfishly'

SHEILA ROWBOTHAM
Women, Resistance and Revolution

Introduction

This handbook has been written for two reasons. Firstly, it aims to help women decide when they should visit the doctor by giving them the basic information about the reproductive and sexual functions of their bodies. It also describes conditions and symptoms related to these functions which require medical advice or attention, such as the need for advice about birth control methods or what to do about a vaginal infection, unusual bleeding or pain in the breasts, genitals or internal pelvic organs. This area of medical specialization is called gynaecology and the doctor who practises it is a gynaecologist. If he also specializes in pregnancy and childbirth he is called an obstetrician.

It describes what to expect in a doctor's surgery and when it may be better to go to a family planning clinic, a well-woman clinic — if you are lucky enough to have one in your area - or to a special clinic (which deals with all types of infection of the sexual organs, not merely those which are transmitted sexually). It explains what the doctor is doing during an internal examination and the appearance and function of the various instruments which he uses. It explains the meaning of unfamiliar medical terms and briefly explains the type of treatment to expect if the doctor makes a particular diagnosis.

Secondly, it aims to improve the relationship between a woman and her doctor by showing both sides how they can understand each other better. It explains why a doctor asks certain questions and what a woman should do, if, as sometimes happens, the right questions are not asked or she feels that she is being treated patronizingly or unsympathetically. It suggests to a woman the information she should be ready to give her doctor and the questions that she should not be too shy to ask.

Use this handbook as a guide to better health care by learning how to talk to your doctor but don't expect it to answer all your questions about the way your body is made and how it functions. It is not intended to be a complete medical manual. That job has already been done several times over and the best of these books are recommended for further reading. You will also find addresses of organizations listed at the end of the handbook.

Throughout the handbook, the doctor is referred to as 'he'. Of course, there are many women doctors in practice and their number is increasing, especially in family planning clinics. However, the fact remains that most obstetricians and gynaecologists are men, as are the majority of general practitioners, and it is more often to a man than to a woman that women patients have to confide some of their most intimate problems.

   This can be a considerable source of embarrassment for a woman and cause her not to explain her case properly. If a woman can learn to talk to her doctor as an equal human being whom she is consulting because he has specialist skills and knowledge to put at her disposal, then we shall have gone a long way to removing the myths and fears which turn doctors either into god-men or enemies.

1 What it feels like to be a woman

One thing every woman knows is that over the years she may have to visit the doctor for many other reasons besides the usual ones of feeling ill or requiring treatment for a particular health condition. This is because for at least forty years of her life, from the onset of menstruation to the time she reaches the menopause, her body is geared to sexuality and reproduction in a way which is not experienced by a man. Nothing can alter this biological fact.

Better methods of birth control, better ante- and post-natal care, constantly developing skills in the management of childbirth, more knowledge about the various conditions arising out of a woman's complex reproductive structure – irrespective of whether or not she has children – and better techniques for treating them, all result from medical advances which have been made in the last fifty years. Unquestionably, they have lightened some of the physical burdens of being a woman, but there is no conceivable scientific technique which could entirely remove the claims made upon a woman's body and mind by her reproductive physiology, nor probably would most women wish this to happen.

A woman uses some of the same organs of her body both for making love and for bearing children. Her breasts may be desired and caressed by her lover, desired and suckled by her child. Her vagina is an important part of love-making as well as being the channel through which she brings her child into the world. Her uterus may respond with spasms of pleasure in orgasm as well as contractions in childbirth.

Many women today enjoy the relatively new freedom of being able to choose whether and when to have children and this has given them the power to separate their sexuality from their reproductive function. This does not mean that they have been turned into sex objects or that they think only of their own sexual gratification. Quite the contrary! The woman who controls her own fertility enhances her own self-esteem. No longer is her sexual life determined by her ovaries.

Yet, in spite of all these advances and the opportunities they offer for happier and more fulfilled lives, many women still feel worried or ashamed about their bodily functions, especially those functions associated with sex. Often we don't care to know too much about what goes on 'down there' and have only a very hazy idea of where our various organs are, how they work or even what they are called. This may be because we have been brought up to think of sex as something a bit dirty, or at any rate something very private which we should keep to ourselves.

Even if we are fairly comfortable with our bodies, it is still quite natural for us to be nervous about the internal examination a doctor may have to give us, particularly if he is a man. The fact that he is wearing a white coat and probably has a nurse in attendance doesn't make it any less of an ordeal. We are being asked to undress, expose ourselves, open our legs and allow a stranger to feel inside our body with a cold instrument which we probably wouldn't recognize if we saw it lying on a table. This makes us feel very vulnerable and invaded and if the doctor is even slightly insensitive, either in the way he handles us or in the way he talks to us, we are likely to react immediately by tensing up physically and feeling too frightened or overawed to ask him the questions we want to put to him.

It may surprise you to know that many doctors are as uneasy and disturbed in this situation as their patients and for this reason often don't do an examination when they should. Doctors are human beings too with their own hang-ups, problems and feelings of inadequacy, but because we think of them as authority figures – a view frequently fostered by doctors themselves because it boosts their self-confidence – we find it hard to imagine that the calm, assured manner, learnt from earliest days in the medical school, may be concealing a frantically worried person, wondering desperately what he should say or what diagnosis he should be making.

As in any other relationship, communication is the key to establishing a good understanding between a woman and her doctor. There are two essential elements for this understanding: each must be prepared to listen to the other and each must be prepared to say honestly and clearly what they think and what they want.

If a doctor, who is supported by his medical knowledge and experience, often finds it difficult to make his meaning clear, then it's hardly surprising that a woman can sometimes find it almost impossible to explain her problem. This is made worse for her if she isn't sure what words to use to describe what she is feeling, whether it be a physical pain or something more elusive like an emotion of distress or worry, or a general impression that something is not quite right with her. Added to this problem about expression is the natural reluctance that most of us feel about revealing secret fears to a stranger. Doctors have been trained to hide their emotions. Women are afraid to show them for fear of looking foolish or being accused of wasting the doctor's time.

Your health is much too important to allow feelings to get in the way of saying what you want to say. If you think you might be too nervous or embarrassed or just plain forgetful when you arrive in the doctor's surgery, spend a little time beforehand jotting down the points you want to make. And don't be afraid to pull out this bit of paper to refer to them if necessary, either before or after you have had your examination.

If the doctor uses words which you don't understand, ask him to repeat what he has said in simpler language. If he prescribes a particular treatment, make sure you know what it is for, and what he hopes to achieve by it. Above all, make sure that the doctor knows why you have come to see him.

To succeed in this, there are certain basic facts about yourself which you must know so that *you* can help the doctor ask you the right questions and *he* can understand why you have come to see him.

2 What every woman must know about herself

A woman's sexual organs are complicated and even those which are on the outside of her body are difficult to see because they are hidden away between her legs.

This illustration shows the position of the female external sex organs and gives the names for the different parts. Look at it carefully. Doctors call this part of a woman's body the *vulva*. Most other people call it the cunt.

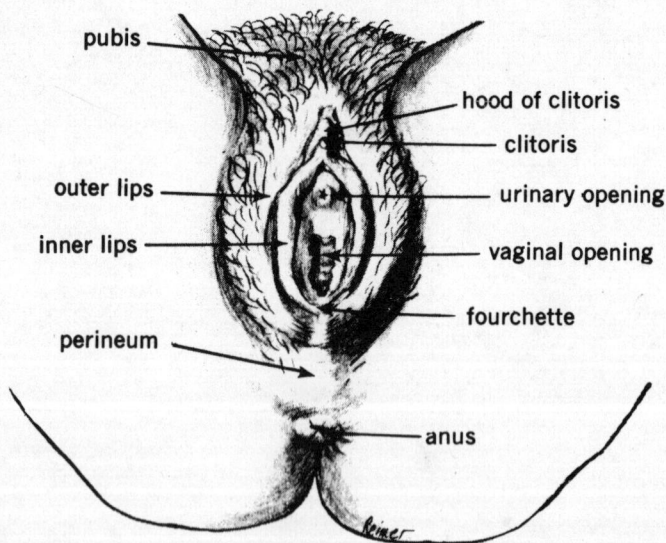

pubis — hood of clitoris — clitoris — outer lips — urinary opening — inner lips — vaginal opening — fourchette — perineum — anus

When you have some time to yourself and know that you won't be disturbed, take off your pants and lie on your bed with your legs bent and your back supported by a pillow. Use a hand mirror to match what you can see of your own body with the illustration.

Pull aside the fleshy outer lips (*labia majora*) so that you can see the thin inner lips (*labia minora*) which surround your vaginal opening and the *urethra* which is the external opening for your bladder. If you are a virgin, you may be able to see a thin layer of skin just inside your vagina. This is called the *hymen* but many girls lose this before they have sexual intercourse, either through using tampons or from doing strenuous exercise. You will see that the labia minora meet in a hood above your vagina. If you press this hood back, your *clitoris* will emerge. This is a small knob of extremely sensitive tissue, similar in some ways to a man's penis, which becomes swollen with blood during sexual excitement and, at the height of stimulation during intercourse or masturbation, produces the sensation of extreme pleasure which is called orgasm.

Many women are concerned about the appearance of their external sex organs. They think there is something wrong with them because they vary in size or shape from pictures which they may have seen, but there is nothing abnormal about this. Just as we all have different faces, so we all have different cunts.

Obviously, a woman can never see her internal reproductive organs because they are contained within the protective cradle of her pelvis. This illustration shows you where they are placed and their relationship to other organs like the bladder and the rectum.

FEMALE REPRODUCTIVE
ORGANS
(SIDE VIEW)

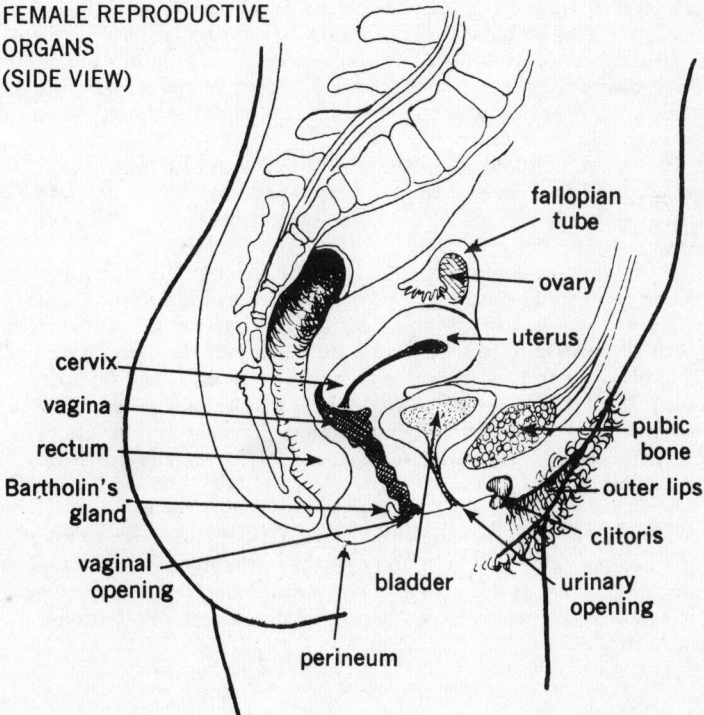

fallopian
tube

ovary

uterus

cervix

vagina

rectum

Bartholin's
gland

pubic
bone

outer lips

clitoris

vaginal
opening

bladder

urinary
opening

perineum

The *uterus* (womb) is a hollow pear-shaped organ about the size of a lemon when it is in a non-pregnant state. The walls of the uterus are very muscular and serve a dual purpose: to protect the growing foetus and to expel the baby, when it is ready to be born, in the strong rhythmic contractions of labour. On either side at the top of the uterus are two hair-like tubes (the *Fallopian tubes*) which are about 4 inches long and widen out at their extremities to curve round the ovaries. Each ovary contains a large store of eggs (*ova*) of which one a month ripens during a woman's reproductive years. When hormonal action releases it from the ovary in the middle of a woman's monthly cycle – this is called *ovulation* – it is drawn into the Fallopian tube by moving fronds at the end of the tube.

The vagina is the passage connecting the uterus to the external sex organs. Think of the vagina as potential space. It is not a rigid hole. It has elastic ridged walls which normally lie in folds touching one another, but which are capable of expanding to accommodate a man's erect penis during intercourse and stretching even more when a baby is being born. At the top end of the vagina, which is approximately 4 to 5 inches long, there is the *cervix* (neck of the womb) which is a blunt shiny knob with a slit in the middle called the *os*. It is through this narrow opening that the man's sperm passes into the uterus to fertilize the woman's egg. It is also capable of stretching wide enough to allow a baby to pass from the uterus to the vagina.

Usually conception does not take place, so each month the lining which has been prepared by the uterus to receive and nourish the fertilized egg breaks away and is washed through the os and down the vagina in the menstrual blood.

If you use tampons, you will be familiar with touching inside your vagina. At a time when you are relaxed, try exploring it with your fingers a little more thoroughly. (Don't forget to wash your hands first.)

If you go deeply enough you can touch your cervix which feels a bit like the tip of your nose. As you draw your fingers out of your vagina you will realize that it is only the last outer third of the vagina which is sensitive to touch because it is here that there are nerve ends. Probably your fingers are wet with a thin, colourless and odourless liquid. The vagina is moist all the time and at certain times becomes very wet, especially during sexual arousal. These secretions are perfectly normal and are a way of cleansing the vagina and protecting it from infection.

Knowing how you are made and knowing the medical names for those parts of your body will help you explain to the doctor why you have come to see him. It will also give you a much better understanding of what he is trying to discover when he asks you certain questions.

3 When a woman should talk to a doctor

There will be many occasions in your life when you need to see a doctor, not necessarily because you are ill but because you need help, advice or information about something to do with your sexual or reproductive life. There will also be times when you do think that there may be something wrong: you may have pain or an unpleasant vaginal discharge or be bleeding outside your normal period. You may want to take preventive measures against the possibility of future disease, for instance by having a smear test for cervical cancer or a breast examination.

You may not always want to go to your family doctor, either for personal reasons or because you think he may not have the specialized knowledge or interest which your particular problem requires. It is important to realize that you do have a choice and that you are *not* obliged to consult your own GP first about everything. For instance, if you are young and unmarried and want to go on the Pill, you may prefer to go to a family planning clinic where the doctors don't know you or your family. Similarly, if you are afraid you may have caught an infection through sexual intercourse, you may prefer to go to one of the special clinics attached to all large hospitals. Here nobody asks you any personal questions – you don't even have to give your name – and you will be treated efficiently if somewhat impersonally. Most doctors in such clinics will avoid moralizing, but just occasionally you may be unlucky and come across one who can't resist making a pointed remark which indicates his disapproval of what he imagines has been your behaviour. All you can do in such circumstances is ignore it, finish your treatment and go to another clinic if you need help again.

The other important point to remember is that you have a right to a second opinion if you are not happy with what your doctor has told you. Many women are frightened to suggest to their doctor that this is what they do want because they think he will be offended and therefore annoyed with them. Sometimes he may be, but that is a risk you will have to take. Remember that your health is always more precious than someone else's hurt feelings so don't be timid about insisting on this right, if you want it. And if you need moral support, then take your boyfriend, a close woman friend, your husband, your mother or anyone else who will be on your side. Two against one is not playing dirty if that one threatens to be a bully.

You have the same right to a second opinion when you are seeing a gynaecologist. (*Gune* is the Greek word for woman and a gynaecologist is a doctor who specializes in treating problems and diseases connected with a woman's reproductive organs). Your GP will give you a letter to see a gynaecologist if he thinks that your problem requires more expert attention than he can give it.

Asking for a second opinion is particularly important if the gynaecologist suggests serious treatment or possibly an operation, without giving you what you consider to be good enough reasons. For instance, he may suggest a *hysterectomy* (removal of the uterus and sometimes the ovaries as well) which will mean that you can no longer have children and, if the ovaries are gone, an early menopause.

As you will see on page 39 there are many good reasons for having a hysterectomy, but it is not unknown for doctors to do this operation quite unnecessarily. In America, where you pay for your health care, the motivation is often quite simple – financial gain. In this country, it is a little more complicated. Doctors who do a lot of hysterectomies will say that they are saving women a lot of trouble and protecting them from the possibility of dangerous disease later on. Others, who are less convinced, observe that the problems sometimes brought on by an artificially induced menopause may be more troublesome than hypothetical cancer.

'Surely you don't want to keep that menstruating uterus now you've completed your family' was the way one doctor put it to a 40 year-old woman who was in hospital with a pelvic infection. Because it wasn't necessary she resisted his almost indecent eagerness to practise his surgical skills and several years later, reports that her uterus is still in excellent working order.

Never accept anything from a doctor just because he is a doctor. He is not God, although he may try to impress you as such, and he does not always know best. Most doctors, however, are genuinely trying to do the best they know how for their patients. You consult a doctor because he has a technical expertise you lack, so hear him out. If he shows impatience when it's your turn to ask the questions, persist tactfully. If you still don't get satisfaction, then insist on a second opinion.

Following is a list of the major reasons which may prompt you to visit the doctor. They have been classified according to whether they refer to a woman in a state of good health, ill health or are matters of prevention rather than cure. Listed next to them are the places or people you can consult and the page numbers indicate where you will find more information about them in this handbook.

'WELL-WOMAN' REASONS

The problem	Who/Where to get help	Page
Menstrual problems	GP who may refer you to a gynaecologist	21 - 23
Contraception	Family Planning Clinic Brook Advisory Centre GP	24 - 32
Pregnancy testing	British Pregnancy Advisory Service (free) Women's Centres Pregnancy Advisory Service Family Planning Clinic Brook Advisory Centre Health Centre GP	34
Pregnancy and childbirth	GP who will refer you to a local hospital if he doesn't handle maternity cases.	35 - 37
Infertility	GP who will refer you to a gynaecologist or a fertility clinic.	33
Abortion	GP for National Health, but if he's not sympathetic, try one of the two charities, BPAS or PAS for low-cost private treatment.	30 - 32
Sterilization	GP who will refer you to a gynaecologist.	29 - 30
Menopause	GP who may refer you to a menopause clinic or to a gynaecologist.	38 - 40
Sexual problems	GP National Marriage Guidance Council Sex Therapist	41

PREVENTIVE REASONS

Breast Examination Cervical Smear Test	GP Well-woman clinic Family planning clinic BUPA (fee) Marie Stopes House (fee)	42 - 43

ILL HEALTH REASONS

The Problem	Who/Where to get help	Page
Vaginal discharge, rash, itching, suspected infection e.g. cystitis, thrush or trichomonal vaginitis (trich). Venereal diseases like syphilis and gonorrhoea caused by having sex with someone who is infected.	GP or Special Clinic at local hospital.	44 - 45
Breakthrough bleeding, pain in breasts, pelvic area or external genitalia. Other abnormalities.	GP who will refer you to a gynaecologist if he suspects there may be something seriously wrong.	

4 What happens when you visit the doctor

The procedure varies, depending on which kind of doctor you are seeing – a GP, a gynaecologist, a family planning specialist, etc. – and for what condition you are consulting him. For example, if all you want is a prescription for a new supply of the pill, he may run through a verbal checklist to make sure that nothing unusual has happened to you between now and your last visit and leave it at that.

However, most of the reasons listed on pages 15/16 which bring a woman to see a doctor, require that she be examined, which means that she will have to undress partially if not completely. Although the details may be different, the following is an outline of the basic procedure.

If it is your first visit, the doctor will ask you questions about your general medical history: what illnesses and operations you may have had, whether you have any allergies and your family background, i.e. whether there is a history of certain illnesses like diabetes or epilepsy. Then he will take a detailed gynaecological history. He will want to know about your menstrual cycle, when you first started menstruation, how regular you are, whether you have any pain, when you had your last period etc. Finally, he will ask you questions which relate specifically to the reason for your visit. For example, if you think you may be pregnant he will want to know the date of your last period, whether you have been pregnant before and whether you have had any miscarriages or other problems.

When you have answered all these questions, you will be asked to undress, taking off your pants and tights if you are to have an internal examination, your top garments as well if the doctor wishes to examine your breasts which he should do. In a clinic, you are given a cubicle in which to undress and hang your clothes, and a gown to wear. In the doctor's surgery you may be able to go behind a screen but sometimes you will be expected to undress in front of him.

He will ask you to climb on to the examining couch, a high, hard, narrow bed which is spread with a clean paper sheet. To do the examination, the doctor will either ask you to lie on your back, draw your legs up and let them fall slightly outwards, or alternatively, he will ask you to turn over on your left side, and bend your legs, one slightly higher than the other. Before doing the internal examination, he will probably but not invariably examine your external sex organs.

The position he asks you to take depends entirely on what he prefers and the way he finds it most comfortable to do an examination. A doctor never asks a woman which way she would like to lie. However, since a good doctor wants to be able to do his examinations as thoroughly and easily as possible, it is to his advantage to make sure that his patient is relaxed, otherwise he will not be able to examine her vagina. For this reason many doctors prefer a woman to lie in the sideways position as they think it is less embarrassing for the patient, and therefore will cause less tension if she does not have to look directly at the doctor during examination.

The doctor will be wearing a rubber glove dipped in KY jelly, which is water soluble and non-sticky and makes it easy for him to slip his two middle fingers into your vagina. Even if you are used to having an internal examination you will probably stiffen unconsciously as he makes his preparations. He will ask you to relax but may not explain how.

The best way to do this is to tighten your vagina a little more and then slowly let your breath out and feel yourself going as limp as possible. Most doctors will do their best to conduct the examination as gently as possible, but if your doctor is a bit rough, then say so. Suffering in silence helps neither him nor you as you will immediately tense up.

First, he will feel round the inside of your vagina; then, still holding your cervix in position with his inserted fingers he will with the fingers of his other hand, press all over the lower part of your abdomen. This is called palpating and the purpose of it is to feel your uterus and the area surrounding it to check that everything is in the right place and that there are no abnormal lumps or bulges indicating possible growths, or inflamed tissue or perhaps a pregnancy. He should be able to feel your ovaries but not your Fallopian tubes unless they are enlarged by a tubal pregnancy (*ectopic* pregnancy) or infection. We will rely on you to tell him where it hurts (if you have been complaining of pain) and how it hurts. It is important that you describe to him as clearly as you can what you are feeling as this will help him with his diagnosis.

When he has finished palpating — this is called the pelvic examination — he will withdraw his fingers from your vagina and insert a speculum to have a closer look at your vagina and cervix.

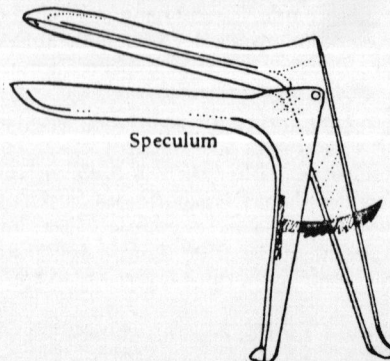

Speculum

A speculum is made either of steel or plastic. It is inserted closed and the two bills are then opened in order to hold the walls of the vagina apart. Providing this is done gently and slowly, you will feel only a minimal discomfort, but tell the doctor immediately if it does hurt. The doctor will shine a strong light up your vagina so that he can see more clearly and he may use an instrument called a *colposcope*, a kind of telescope which magnifies the cervix. What he will be checking for are the colour, texture and appearance of your vagina and cervix, and the colour, smell and consistency of your vaginal secretions.

It is quite normal for a healthy woman's vagina and cervix to change colour at various times in her menstrual cycle – anything from pale pink to deep purplish blue – and her vaginal secretions will also vary in consistency depending on her oestrogen level. Pregnancy also produces a marked change in colour but the doctor will be looking for abnormal discolourations and changes in shape.

He may take a cervical smear to check for early signs of cancer and/or your oestrogen level, particularly important if you are approaching menopause. To do this he uses a wooden spatula to scrape a few cells off your cervix and probably inserts a cotton-tipped applicator or pipette to take a sample of vaginal secretion. This sounds nasty but if it's done carefully it's painless as the cervix is a fairly insensitive organ. It feels more like a tickle than a scratch. Occasionally, he may decide to do a rectovaginal examination as well which means that he inserts one finger into your rectum (back passage) and the other into your vagina. This is usually done if he can't find the ovaries by ordinary palpatation or he suspects disease of some kind.

When he has finished his examination he will ask you to get off the couch. If you have to get dressed in his presence, do so before you ask any questions. Anyway, always wait until you are either sitting or standing before you ask him questions as this restores you to a position of equality. Remember, if he says anything you don't understand, ask him to repeat it in plainer language. Sometimes, there is little he can say until the results of tests he may also have made have come back from the laboratory.

In subsequent sections we shall be describing in more detail the kind of questions you should ask and how, in different situations.

No woman enjoys having an internal examination, but it is very often vitally necessary. Some doctors don't like doing them, because they have mixed feelings about touching their women patients. They are afraid of the sexual connotations and some doctors are genuinely afraid that a woman may leap off the couch and make unbridled amorous advances. Very rarely indeed this does occur but most women feel anything but sexy in what is invariably a somewhat undignified and humbling situation. If you think you should have an examination and your doctor refuses to give you one, ask for a second opinion. Often a doctor affects a blustering or patronizing manner to hide his own embarrassment, or he develops mannerisms as a protective shell so that his patients cannot guess at his own unease.

Not all examinations are conducted in the way described above. There are some old-fashioned hospitals where women are still asked to sling their legs into overhead stirrups for an internal examination. This is not necessary and it certainly doesn't help to relax you. If you are faced with this situation, there is nothing much you can do about it at the time except to shut your eyes and remember that nothing lasts forever. However, if you do strongly dislike this method, say so afterwards to the doctor. Ask him why he uses this approach and if his answer doesn't satisfy you make it plain how you feel about it. If enough women raised objections it would force doctors to reconsider their practises.

Sometimes a woman who is being examined in a clinic attached to a teaching hospital may find that her doctor has invited some of his medical students to watch. Do you know that you are entitled to refuse the hospital this facility? It may be more difficult if the doctor asks one or more people to come and have a look during the examination and you would need to be exceptionally strong-minded – or angry — to jump off the couch there and then. However, this privacy is your right and if you have any fears that it might be disregarded, ask for a written undertaking beforehand.

5 Menstrual problems

The average age at which girls start to menstruate is between 12 and 14, but it can be normal to start as early as 9 or as late as 17. It is a sign that their ovaries are now functioning and producing ripe eggs, usually alternatively and in a monthly cycle. This is called ovulation and if the egg is not fertlized it will pass through the cervix unnoticed a few days after ovulation. Menstruation, which happens about two weeks later, is the process by which the uterus discards the lining it has prepared to receive a fertilized egg. The duration of the menstrual flow varies with individual women from 2 to 8 days and is called a period.

The majority of girls and women will experience some sort of menstrual problem in their reproductive life, but because we are brought up not to make a fuss about minor aches and pains we usually try to ignore them unless they become intolerable. You should consult your doctor if you have any of the following difficulties.

PROLONGED IRREGULARITY

Minor irregularities are quite normal. A woman will quite probably have varying lengths of cycle within a year and if she suffers illness, emotional shock or stress her periods may come on early or late. Young girls sometimes have irregular periods while their menstrual cycle is establishing itself.

If your menstrual cycle is repeatedly irregular you should see your doctor as it may mean you have a hormonal imbalance which is affecting your ovulation. Some doctors put women on the Pill to establish regularity, because it automatically makes a 28-day cycle. This may not be wise if you are very young (under 19) and have not yet given your body a chance to establish its own rhythm.

If your doctor suggests the Pill for this reason, ask him to explain how he expects it to work for you.

PAIN (DYSMENORRHOEA)

Spasmodic This is sharp stomach cramps in the lower abdomen, sometimes accompanied by nausea and shivering. This usually happens to young women between the ages of 15 and 25 and invariably disappears with pregnancy and childbirth. If pain relievers, hot water bottles, gentle exercise or rest are not enough to ease the pain, consult your doctor. Swimming, baths, washing your hair, etc., do not affect your periods.

He may suggest the Pill, but make sure that he understands the kind of pain you are having as some pills actually cause worse pain. This is because they contain too much of the wrong hormone for your condition. Spasmodic dysmenorrhoea means that you are producing excessive progesterone compared with oestrogen, so a high oestrogen pill may help but it does have other disadvantages (see page 26) and it may not be wise to continue it for too long.

Doctors have been known to say, 'What you need, my dear, is a baby'. This is flippant, irresponsible and objectionable and you should make it clear to him that you think so in whatever way suits you best: a cold stare or a remark to the effect that you don't believe in having babies for your own or other people's convenience.

Congestive This is a nagging pain in the lower abdomen, backache, a general feeling of lethargy and discomfort which often starts several days before the period and is only relieved when the period is fully established. It is frequently accompanied by other symptoms such as swollen breasts and stomach, caused by water retention, headache, aching joints and depression which is collectively known as *premenstrual tension.* This type of pain can last through a woman's reproductive life, but as it is due to excess oestrogen it can be treated with progesterone, a natural hormone. A high dosage progestogen is *not* suitable for this condition as progestogen is a synthetic, i.e. artificially manufactured hormone and actually reduces the level of progesterone.

If your doctor does not understand this important distinction, refer him to Dr Katharine Dalton's book, *The Menstrual Cycle* (Penguin 1970).

Many doctors, including some women doctors, and nurses who are lucky enough not to suffer from period problems, are inclined to pooh-pooh those women who do complain of serious discomfort. If your doctor is unsympathetic, ask for a second opinion. It is not worth living with unnecessary pain to satisfy other people's prejudices.

LACK OF PERIODS (AMENORRHOEA)

This is *primary* if a girl hasn't started menstruating by the age of 18 and *secondary* if a woman's periods cease at any time after starting. It may happen because she isn't ovulating, or is suffering from stress, illness or a congenital defect. Always consult your doctor if this happens to you.

HEAVY OR UNEXPECTED BLEEDING

Some women naturally have a heavier and more prolonged blood flow. If they are fitted with an IUD (see page 26) this is inevitable. They should however, guard against iron deficiency (*anaemia*) which will make them feel listless and possibly make them more prone to infection.

If you suddenly start to bleed more heavily than usual or it happens at other times of the month (*breakthrough bleeding*) consult your doctor because it is almost certainly an indication that there is something wrong with your internal reproductive organs – not necessarily serious, but whatever it is, it should be attended to.

6 Birth control — which method?

If you are having sex and you don't want to become pregnant, you must use some form of birth control. Ideally, you will discuss it with your man beforehand and together decide on the method which suits you both best. If for some reason this is difficult for you to do, then the responsibility lies entirely with you. You are the person who will be landed with an unwanted pregnancy, so it is up to you to inform yourself and choose whatever suits you best.

Sometimes this is easier said than done. Although family planning advice and supplies are now given free to men and women as part of the National Health Service, many GPs are not particularly interested in this aspect of their practice. Alternatively, they may 'push' one method without sufficiently explaining the other types. You may have personal reasons for not wanting to discuss birth control with your doctor, for instance, if you are unmarried and you fear his disapproval.

If you can, it is probably better to go to a family planning clinic run by the health department of your local authority or to a voluntary organization like the Brook Advisory Centre. (Addresses at the end of the book or look up Family Planning in the telephone book).

In these clinics the doctors are specially trained to do family planning and they will give you the time and confidentiality you need to choose what is best for you. Don't make up your mind in a hurry. Read the leaflets which you can pick up at any of these clinics, but remember they only explain the various methods. They don't tell you about possible side effects. For complete information read some of the books mentioned in this handbook.

There are three main points that you should consider when comparing the relative merits of the different methods:

1. **Reliability** i.e. how likely is it to prevent conception?
2. **Safety** i.e. does it have any side effects which could damage your health?
3. **Convenience** i.e. is it easy to use? does it suit your particular way of life? does it appeal to you personally as a method?

Use this RSC test to help you decide which method you are going to choose, but remember that *no* contraceptive has yet been produced which is perfect in all these respects. You will have to make a compromise of some sort. Choose what suits you best, which may not be the same as the doctor recommends. Remember too that during the course of your life, your needs, your health and your circumstances will change, so be prepared to be flexible.

Below are listed only those methods which require a visit to the doctor.

THE PILL (ORAL CONTRACEPTIVE)

There are three types now in use:

The combination pill containing synthetic versions of the female hormones of oestrogen and progesterone. This pill works by preventing ovulation i.e. the egg does not ripen in the ovary and is therefore, not released. It is taken once a day for the first 21 days of the menstrual cycle, starting on the 5th day after menstruation begins.

The sequential pill is also taken for 21 days but the first 14 pills contain oestrogen only, the last 7 a combination of both oestrogen and progestogen. Works by preventing ovulation but not used so much now as it's not thought to be as effective as the combination pill.

The continuous or **mini pill** contains progestogen only and works by thickening the cervical mucus, therefore acting as a barrier to sperm and it also changes the lining of the uterus. However, it doesn't always prevent ovulation and so is not quite as reliable as the Combination Pill. It is taken throughout the menstrual cycle, in other words, for 28 days.

This is how the pill scores on the RSC test:

Reliability – almost 100 per cent in theory, but about 2 per cent actual failure, due probably to forgetting it or not backing it up by another method, either when starting it or changing to another brand.

Safety – different pills have different effects on different women. You may have to try several brands before you find the right one for you, which means the one which has the least side effects. The reason for this variation is that we all have different hormone levels. Less serious side effects include weight gain, nausea, headaches, depression, thrush, skin problems.

More serious ones include thrombosis, migraine, liver tumours, hypertension and gall stones.

The Pill is now known in certain cases to increase susceptibility to strokes, VD, urinary tract infection, diabetes, epilepsy and certain forms of cancer.

The Pill is only available on prescription and women should resist the efforts being made to have it available in supermarkets and the like. We still have not seen a whole generation go through their

entire cycle on the Pill and we still don't know everything we need
to know about it. If you decide to go on the Pill you should be given
a thorough medical examination which will include: a medical case
history with the doctor checking for high blood pressure, migraine,
diabetes, varicose veins, epilepsy, in yourself and your family. This
should be followed by a careful physical examination including
breasts, pelvic, urine and smear test. Make sure that you do get all
this the first time and that thereafter you have an annual medical
check-up, more frequently if you suffer from migraine, diabetes,
asthma, epilepsy, varicose veins or are over 35.

Women who should not take the Pill are those who have had any
form of cancer, liver disease or are subject to conditions of blood
circulation or excess blood clotting. It is definitely inadvisable over
the age of 40. Doctors are still divided about whether there should
be a time limit on using the Pill. Some advise coming off it after two
or three years of continuous use; others take the view that if the
woman herself feels perfectly all right then that is the best test of
the Pill. The truth is that no one really knows. However, one thing
is certain. A woman's fertility is often affected for a short period
after coming off the Pill until her ovaries start functioning normally
again, so don't expect to get pregnant in a hurry.

Convenience – Against these side effects must be set the convenience of not having to insert anything, although you do have to remember to take your pill.

DEPO-PROVERA (INJECTABLE CONTRACEPTIVE)

This is based on the same hormonal principle as the Pill but it can
be given by injection once every three or six months. About one
million women are currently on this method, mainly in developing
countries, but it has been officially banned in the USA and this
country. Nonetheless a lot of doctors are prescribing it. Measured
on the RSC test Depo-provera scores high on Reliability and Convenience, but badly on Safety. These are some of the side effects
it may cause: irregular or prolonged menstruation, headaches, depression, weight gain, vomiting and rectal bleeding. It has been
proved to have links with infertility, blood clotting and is suspected
to have a connection with breast and cervical cancer. Avoid this
method.

THE IUD (INTRA-UTERINE DEVICE OFTEN KNOWN AS THE COIL OR LOOP)

This is a small plastic or metal device which is inserted into the
uterus during or just after a period when the cervix is soft and open.
It can only be put there, and removed, by a doctor who has been
specially trained. Some GPs have had this training – you can check

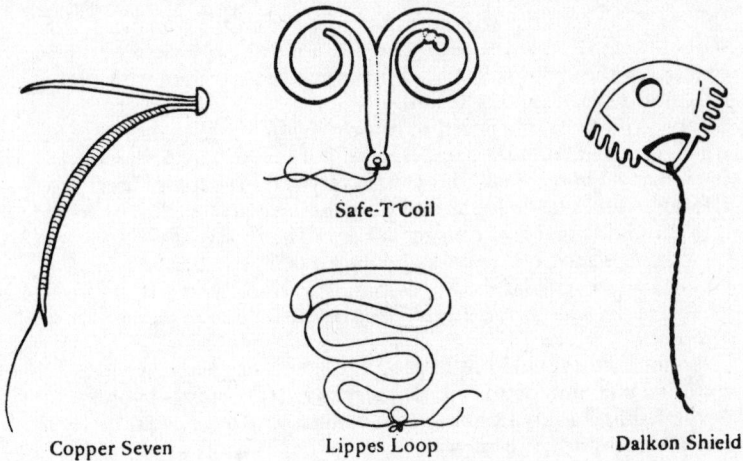

Safe-T-Coil

Copper Seven   Lippes Loop   Dalkon Shield

this by ringing your local Family Practitioner Committee – and all family planning doctors have had it. It has been shown that insertions done by trained doctors considerably reduce the risk of complications. A small string is attached to the coil which comes through the os into the vagina and a woman should check for herself at least once a month (best after her period) to make sure that it is still there.

No one is quite sure how the IUD prevents conception but it probably happens by preventing the egg from implanting itself into the wall of the uterus.

The types of IUD used are Lippes Loop and Safe-T-Coil for women who have had children and who therefore have a slightly enlarged uterus. The Copper 7 and Copper T are for women who have not had a pregnancy. These both have copper wound round the stem.

Ask your doctor what type of IUD he intends inserting into you. Ask to see it and ask him to explain why he thinks he has chosen the best type for you. Don't accept the Dalkon Shield. It has been banned in America and many doctors here now don't use it either, because it has been shown to cause severe problems of bleeding, infection, etc.

This is how the IUD scores on the RSC test:

Reliability — second only to the pill, with a failure rate of about 1.7 per cent providing that it is not expelled by the uterus, (usually within the first three months by about 10 per cent of women) and that you can stand it. However, about 25 per cent of women find that it causes pain or heavy bleeding which they find intolerable. Its effectiveness may be diminished if you are taking aspirin or antibiotics, so if reliability is essential then it's wise to use extra contraceptives at that time, e.g. foam, cream, jelly or condom, all of which are available over the counter without prescription from the chemist. If you should become pregnant with the IUD, removing it makes it 50 per cent likely that you will have a miscarriage. Babies born with the IUD still in place are unaffected.

Safety — the IUD is believed to cause a low-lying pelvic infection which may suddenly flare up, especially if you catch another infection, e.g. gonorrhoea. This can be very serious because it can affect the tubes (*salpingitis*) and cause permanent sterility, or spread into the abdominal area causing pelvic inflammatory disease.

Warning signs: if you have abdominal pain, swelling or pain on intercourse, go and see the doctor. Occasionally, the IUD can perforate the wall of the uterus. This is usually due to clumsy insertion.

Women who should not have an IUD are those who have had a uterine infection or an ectopic pregnancy (conception in one of the Fallopian tubes), nor should women who have cysts, fibroids or erosion of the cervix.

Convenience — once in, the IUD can stay put for 2 to 3 years, subject to annual medical check-ups. However, a woman should check for herself once a month that it is still in place. This can be done in the bath or simply by squatting and inserting your finger the way you would put in a tampon and feeling for the string which dangles into your vagina.

DIAPHRAGM (DUTCH CAP)

This is a dome-shaped soft rubber cap with a spring inside the rim which holds it in place over the cervix. It acts as a barrier preventing the sperm from entering the uterus.

You have to be measured for a diaphragm by the doctor according to the width of your upper vagina. When he does the fitting he will also show you how to insert it, but if you have any doubts or problems, don't hesitate to ask him. That's what he's there for.

Before inserting it, spread spermicidal cream or jelly over the inside of the dome and round the rim. This is very important because the cap on its own is not sufficient. Then press the cap into an oval shape with your thumb and forefinger, push it high up your vagina, behind your pubic bone and release the spring. It will then be covering your cervix.

It should be left in place for at least 8 hours after intercourse and when you remove it, wash and dry it, checking for holes. Caps need to be replaced about once a year.

This is how the diaphragm scores on the RSC test:

Reliability – depends very much on the user. It's not reliable at all without the back up of spermicides but with them and providing that it's not put in more than 2 to 3 hours beforehand and not

taken out too quickly, and the spermicide renewed if intercourse
takes place again, then it has a failure rate of as low as 2.4 per cent
but that is a lot of ifs and buts.
Safety – absolutely no side effects whatsoever unless you produce
an allergic reaction to the spermicide.
Convenience – depends how you view it. If you can train yourself
to make it a habit, like brushing your teeth, then it can become
quite easy. However, it does need a bit of practice and fiddling
around with creams or, putting it in before you feel in the mood
to make love may be very off-putting. Some couples find it helps
to overcome the off-putting aspect by having the man help the
woman to insert it.

STERILIZATION

You may decide that you don't want any more children. If you are
married and already have a family this is obviously a matter which
you will first discuss with your husband unless you have very special reasons for not wishing to do so. It may be that your doctor
will advise you to be sterilized for health reasons. Some women
will decide that they don't want children under any circumstances.
These women will find it very difficult to get a sterilization. Yet
there are other occasions when a doctor will suggest sterilization
to a woman who doesn't want it, for instance, as a condition of
giving her an abortion. Although doctors are very good at telling
women what they should and should not do, especially as far as
motherhood is concerned, they are not so good about listening to
women's views and reasons. The decision whether to have children
at all, or to stop having them rests with you. Although most doctors
will ask your husband to sign a form of consent and the same is
done when a man has a vasectomy, this has no legal force. It is not
required by law and it is done, really, to protect the doctors from
an irate spouse. However, it is a fact that many doctors will refuse
to do the operation unless your husband signs this form. Remember,
sterilization is irreversible. You can't change your mind therefore;
if you want it, you have to be as cool and rational as possible when
producing arguments.

How sterilization is done

There are two possible methods. The first involves an 8 to 10 day
stay in hospital. The second can be an out-patient procedure although in fact most doctors prefer their patients to stay in over-
night.

Tubal Ligation — under a general anaesthetic, the doctor makes an
incision in the abdomen, cuts each Fallopian tube, ties the ends, and

then folds them back into the surrounding tissue. This can also be done through the vagina but is more difficult.

Laparoscopy — a minute incision is made either through the abdomen or less usually through the vagina. An instrument called a laparascope which is a light at the end of a telescope is pushed through to light up the Fallopian tubes which are then cauterized (burnt) by an electric current passed through forceps which come through another minute incision. The advantage of this method is that recovery time is much shorter and scarring is almost nil. However, it does need a skilled, experienced doctor because if he doesn't know exactly what he is doing he may burn the wrong tissue.

If your doctor is not keen to do a laparoscopy then don't press him. He probably won't do it at all well but you can ask for a second opinion or ask him to recommend you to a doctor who will and can do the operation.

ABORTION

This comes under the general heading of birth control because that is precisely what it is, but obviously it should be looked upon as a last resort, a back-up measure when whatever form of contraception you have been using has failed. At the present time the 1967 Act is still in force which means that a woman can have an abortion provided that she has the signed consent of two doctors who agree that her physical or mental health will be affected or that her living or social conditions, e.g. bad housing or too many children already, will seriously impair the future of this new child.

Abortion is a very emotional issue, hence the strong lobbies both in favour of it and against it. In 1975 and again in 1977 two bills have been brought up in Parliament (James White and William Benyon) seeking to restrict the present provisions. Neither have been successful but if an Act similar to these is passed women will be back in the position they were before the 1967 Act and back-street, i.e. illegal, abortions will again happen on a large scale.

If your doctor is against abortion he has every right under the present Act to refuse to give his consent. However, *you* have the right to ask him to recommend you to another doctor for a second opinion. If he refuses to do this as well, then you have no choice but to seek another doctor on your own. It may be necessary for you to consider having an abortion privately. The arguments that a doctor will use to talk you out of your decision run as follows: you don't really know what you want; naturally at the moment you feel frightened and confused but once you have the baby in your arms you will feel pleased and grateful. If he's religious he will say that abortion is murder and that God will provide.

He may not be straightforward. Having made it clear that he

disapproves of you for having asked for an abortion and perhaps suggested that promiscuity merits punishment, he may then agree reluctantly to arrange for an abortion but take his time about it. Beware this approach as it could endanger your health. Abortions done within the first three months by the vacuum aspiration method (explained below) are actually safer than childbirth, but the longer an abortion is delayed, the more complicated the procedure and the more risks you run.

If you do come up against a stone wall about getting an abortion, then your only course is to refer to one of the charities listed at the end of the book. If you find it impossible to raise the money immediately for the abortion (now about £70) they may be able to help you with an interest-free loan.

Methods of abortion

Vacuum Aspiration – this is the safest and preferred method which can be done between 7 and 12 weeks when the pregnancy is con- firmed.

The cervix is first gently dilated to approximately the width of a finger. Then a flexible plastic tube is inserted into the uterus through the cervix and the other end is attached to a machine which is then turned on to suck out the contents of the womb. This takes between 2 to 5 minutes and can be done under local anaesthetic. Sometimes a doctor will follow this up by scraping round the womb with a curette – a small spoon-shaped instru- ment – to make sure that nothing has been left behind in the womb. If done under local anaesthetic in an out-patient clinic, the woman will then rest for about an hour before being allowed to go home. You may have some cramps and minor bleeding for a few days afterwards, but unless they are serious there is no need to call a doctor. Your period will come back within 2 to 4 weeks.

Dilation and Curettage – done between the 12th and 15th week. This is a minor operation requiring general anaesthetic. The cer- vix is dilated and the contents of the uterus scraped loose and removed with forceps. This can also be done for other condi- tions like fibroids but it is more traumatic, i.e. causes more shock to the uterus and that is why you should expect to have to stay in hospital for at least one night, possibly longer.

Induced labour — there are various methods for inducing in later pregnancy what amounts to a miscarriage, usually from 16 to 20 weeks. Either some of the amniotic fluid is drawn off from the uterus and replaced by a mixture of salts and water which causes contractions and eventually miscarriage several hours later or prostaglandins (a type of hormone) are introduced either through the mouth or intravenously. These are generally considered to be safer and labour is induced faster. This is a painful method as it is in effect a mini-labour and you are giving birth to a recognizable child so it is also more emotionally distressing.

Hysterotomy – is a mini-Caesarian involving major surgery. The wall of the abdomen is cut through and the foetus removed. It does not affect future fertility but it may mean that pregnancies carried to full term will have to be done by Caesarian.

Obviously, from every point of view it is advisable that you have your abortion, once you have decided upon it, as soon as possible.

7 You want a baby

Maybe you have been trying to get pregnant for some months, possibly even a year or two. You have given up using any method of birth control and yet you find that nothing happens. You shouldn't let this go on for more than six months. If this is your problem then you must seek the advice of your doctor. He will be able to give you an examination to establish firstly that there is nothing physically abnormal about you which prevents full intercourse and, therefore, the sperm from getting up to your uterus, and secondly, that you are ovulating properly.

In the past if a woman couldn't get pregnant it was she who was held responsible for her barrenness. Today we know better but only a little better. One out of ten couples are infertile and it may be due to more than one cause. Infertility may be caused by physical weakness in the woman or it may be that the man is producing too little sperm or abnormal ones. Her cervical fluids may be killing his sperm. They may not be making love in a way which ensures full penetration. Roughly speaking, one third of infertile marriages are due to the woman, one third to the man and the remaining third are a combination of causes common to both.

If you think that your doctor is treating your problem too lightly — for instance, he may say to take a holiday, relax, or try a bit harder, all of which may seem quite humorous to him but not to you – don't accept what he says. Explain that it matters to both you and your husband and that on the whole you feel it should be treated as a technical problem, not a magic/psychological one. Therefore, could he either send you to a doctor specializing in fertility or to one of the many clinics now operating side by side with family planning clinics. It is very important that your husband joins you in this as you will both have to have tests and be examined. It is important to find a doctor who is *interested* in infertility. Some doctors just aren't; they're interested in fertility and pregnancies, childbirth, etc. People who have had experience say that doctors concerned with the specific problem of infertility are likely to be more sympathetic and more knowledgeable about what can be done.

There are a number of tests which can be done but not all of them are necessary for everyone. Look at *The New Women's Health Handbook,* edited by Nancy MacKeith (Virago 1978) for a clear explanation of them. Incidentally, this book is a good source of further information on most of the topics discussed in this handbook.

8 You want to know whether you are pregnant

There are some classic signs which indicate that you are probably pregnant such as not having your period for more than two weeks after the due date; a sudden urge to pass water more frequently and perhaps a feeling of tenderness and enlargement in your breasts. Whether or not you have been pregnant before, you cannot be sure until you have a test or are examined by your doctor, or both.

Testing is now very simple and you can buy a do-it-yourself home kit. However, if you want to be 100 per cent sure, and most women do, it is better to go either to a family planning clinic or to your GP for the test. The advantage of many clinics, particularly those run by women's groups, is that they will do it for nothing and tell you the results immediately, whereas a doctor will send away your urine sample and this may mean waiting up to 10 days for the result — too long if you think you may want an abortion should the result be positive (look at *The Women's Directory* by Carolyn Faulder, Christine Jackson and Mary Lewis (Virago 1976) for a country-wide list of women's groups).

Pregnancy testing on urine is 95 per cent accurate if it is done after 40 days of pregnancy. If the results are positive, then the doctor will have to confirm them by doing an internal examination. The cervix goes a bluish colour during pregnancy and he will also palpate your abdomen (described on page 18) to see whether your uterus is enlarged.

9 You are pregnant and you want to keep your baby

If you have made this decision, then it is very important both for your own sake and for the health of your unborn child that you take full advantage of the ante-natal care which is available on the National Health Service.

If your GP specializes in maternity cases, then you would probably be well advised to stick with him as he is likely to take a special interest in your progress. If he does not, then he will introduce you to the local hospital.

At the beginning of your pregnancy you will have a thorough medical examination — rather like the check-ups described on page 17 but even more detailed because it is important that if there are going to be any difficulties or complications they should be spotted now. Many women sail through pregnancy relatively easily; some positively blossom, especially after the first three months when nausea ceases and their body has become accustomed to its new condition. Some however do meet difficulties.

For the first seven months of pregnancy your doctor will expect to see you once a month. However, if you have any unusual symptoms like bleeding or pain, you must see him immediately as this may indicate a threatened miscarriage.

On the first visit you will be given a blood test to check that you have no diseases, e.g. syphilis, and to establish your blood type, important if you turn out to be *Rhesus negative* as this could be incompatible with your baby's blood: a urine test to check for kidney and diabetic disease: blood pressure is taken at every visit to make sure that you are not suffering from *hypertension* or *toxaemia:* internal examinations will continue to be done to check that the growth and position of the baby is correct.

There are other tests which can be done later in pregnancy to check for abnormalities like mongolism and spina bifida but they are not done automatically.

After the seventh month you will be seeing your doctor or visiting the ante-natal clinic once a fortnight and then, once you have reached the ninth month, weekly until your labour starts.

It is very important to know as much as you can beforehand about what to expect when you are in labour. One of the best ways of doing this is to attend ante-natal classes and learn to do the exercises, the relaxation and the breathing which will help you during labour.

However, the process of childbirth has become increasingly mechanized in the last few years and many women find that they are treated as objects rather than human beings at this time, both by doctors and nurses. *Induction*, which is the artificial stimulation of labour by means of a hormonal drip, and *epidural* delivery, which is the anaesthetizing of the lower part of the body by means of a spinal injection to ensure painless but conscious birth, can be boons, but only when they are done for the sake of the mother's health and that of her baby. You have a right to refuse them if you suspect that they are being done for the convenience of the doctor and the hospital staff. Make sure that you understand about these and other procedures connected with childbirth, by reading up about them and discussing them with your doctor and your ante-natal tutor. You must ask the doctor *why* he recommends induction, or other procedures, and you have the right to reject his recommendation if you don't think that it is justified on medical grounds, or ask for a second opinion. This can be difficult, especially if the doctor makes a great show of being pressed for time or treats you as if you were a baby machine rather than an adult person with a mind of their own, but it's worth insisting, even if you do run the risk of being branded as neurotic or hysterical. Women must become braver and protest more, if the circumstances warrant it, because until they do, the medical profession will continue to do what *it* thinks best without reference to the people who matter most — the patients.

After you have had your baby, you will find that it takes a bit of time to get adjusted to this new and very demanding presence in your life, particularly if this is your first baby, and just at a time when you need double the energy to cope with the sleepless nights, the endless feeding demands, the constant changing and washing of clothes, you may perhaps feel at your most listless and lethargic, possibly very depressed. You may be frightened by the strong waves of anti-maternal feeling which sweep over you.

Nowadays much more is known about post-natal depression than even five years ago and doctors are at least more sympathetic though they may not be much better at handling it. A bottle of tranquillizers really is not the answer.

If you are frightened by your strong feelings talk to your doctor and tell him what is happening. If he says that all young mothers suffer occasionally from fits of the baby blues, point out that while you are aware of this, what you want to know is how to deal with them. It may be that you need a good rest, possibly a holiday with your husband if you can find a willing and capable grandmother or friend with whom to leave the baby, or if this is not possible, then just the opportunity to talk out how you feel with someone sympathetic.

Six weeks after the birth you must visit your doctor with your baby. He will give you a post-natal examination to make sure that you are not suffering from excessive bleeding and that you have no infection or other problem. He will also examine the baby to make sure that it is normal, but after this it is still a good thing to go to your health clinic fairly regularly for advice on feeding, any injections that may be necessary and generally have a chance to discuss your baby's progress.

However, don't expect the doctor or the health visitor to know everything about *your* child. Views on child-rearing change all the time and some of them are based on fads rather than facts. If you are worried about your child or don't agree with the advice that you have been given, say so, giving your reasons. If you think that you have serious cause for concern which the doctor is not taking seriously, ask for a second opinion.

10 You are starting the change of life

When a women in her mid to late forties finds that her periods are beginning to be erratic — perhaps she misses a month or one month her period is light and the next time it is delayed and very heavy — she will guess that she is beginning the menopause. Should she have other symptoms as well, sudden drenching sweats known as hot flushes (or flashes), itching in her genitals and a feeling of dryness in her vagina, then she will know quite definitely that she is menopausal.

The menopause means that a woman has reached the end of her reproductive life. Her pituitary gland stops producing the hormones which stimulate egg production (*ovulation*) and her ovaries stop producing the hormones *oestrogen* and *progesterone* which change and thicken the lining of the uterus in preparation for the fertilized egg. When this happens, she ceases to menstruate and after a year of having no periods she can be certain that she is no longer fertile. A few women go through the menopause in their thirties, a few as late as sixty, but for most of us it happens round the age of fifty.

The menopause is a different experience for each woman. For some women their periods will stop, perhaps quite suddenly, and that is the beginning and end of it. For others, the menopause may last for as long as five years and may be accompanied by quite a number of other symptoms such as palpitations, dizziness, headaches, moodiness, insomnia and depression. How much these are due to the physical fact of the menopause, and the disturbed hormonal balance it induces, and how much to the individual woman's feelings about the menopause is difficult to resolve.

While it is true to say that the menopause marks the end of one stage of your life — never again will you be able to have a child — it is certainly not the end of your sexual life. Indeed, many women find that sex becomes much more enjoyable after the menopause just because they are freed from the fear of pregnancy. Although not nearly enough research has yet been done into the psychological effects of menopause, it does seem that women who have fulfilled and interesting lives with plenty to occupy them outside their home and family commitments are less likely to be seriously upset by the menopause.

However, no woman entirely escapes the physical changes which are caused by the drop in oestrogen output. If the loss is sudden, then she will experience the hot flushes, and itching, usually round the vulva, but sometimes all over her body, already mentioned. The flushes manifest themselves by an embarrassing colouring-up of the face and neck followed by sweating and can happen quite unexpectedly at any time of the day and night. Genital itching is uncomfortable and a dry vagina — another common symptom — can make intercourse very painful.

Don't suffer these symptoms in silence because they can be dealt with by a straightforward course of oestrogen replacement, in the form of tablets, injections or creams and ointments. Explain your problem to your doctor but if he doesn't seem interested, knowledgeable or sympathetic, then ask for a second opinion. Many hospitals now have a menopause clinic and for a complete list of them, together with names of doctors specializing in menopausal problems, send a stamped addressed envelope to Women's Health Care, address at the end of the book.

Hormone replacement therapy, as this treatment is called, or HRT for short, can be short term or long term. Many doctors are willing to prescribe it for these obvious menopausal symptoms for a limited period of time, but are dubious about the benefits of continuous therapy to counteract the long-term effects of oestrogen loss, which are suffered to a greater or lesser degree by all women. These manifest themselves in the following signs of ageing: loss of muscle and skin tone leading to sagging breasts, flabbiness in the pelvic muscles and wrinkles; thinning of the vaginal wall; sparse, lifeless hair; growth of facial hair and eventually a decrease of calcium causing brittle bones and possibly a curved spine known as 'dowager's hump'. The reason for their caution is that there is some evidence from America, where hormone replacement therapy has been widely used for many years, which links it with breast and uterine cancer in older women.

It is, therefore, very important that if you do want HRT you should discuss it with a doctor who fully understands the pros and cons. Dosage has to be carefully measured and monitored on an individual basis as women vary in their oestrogen levels. Some, for instance, lose much less oestrogen than others in their post-menopausal life because other organs in their body produce the hormone.

An artificial menopause is caused by having your ovaries removed surgically. This may be done as part of a total hysterectomy, an operation in which uterus and Fallopian tubes are also removed, or it is done (rarely) on its own, usually because of disease. The oestrogen loss this causes is usually remedied by an oestrogen implant or injections.

Generally speaking, hysterectomies are performed for good reasons. You may have fibroids which are non-malignant growths in the uterus, causing pain and heavy bleeding as well as a greatly enlarged uterus. You may have cancer in which case there really is no alternative to surgery. You may have severe menstrual irregularities for which, if you are over 40 and don't want any more children, a hysterectomy is the best solution. However, as was pointed out on page 14, doctors sometimes advise a hysterectomy for convenience rather than medical reasons. If your doctor gives you good reasons such as those mentioned above, accept them, but if he is hesitant or doesn't convince you, then ask for a second opinion.

A hysterectomy does not affect your enjoyment of sex, but it is a major operation which will leave you feeling weak for some time afterwards. You may also feel depressed and unhappy, particularly if you don't understand what the operation involves or are not sure what the surgeon has taken out. Ask him to explain beforehand exactly what he intends to do and discuss possible after effects. You will have to sign a form before the operation which authorizes him to remove whatever organs he thinks are necessary, including your ovaries. Ask him afterwards exactly what he has done. Some doctors do this anyway, but don't be afraid to insist if he shows any reluctance. Full knowledge is your absolute right.

11 Your sex life is unsatisfactory

What can you do about it? Perhaps it is years since you have experienced an orgasm, or possibly you never have. You wonder if there is something wrong with you because you seldom or never feel aroused by love-making. You worry because you find that you can climax quite easily when you masturbate but not when you make love. On all sides you hear and read about how wonderful sex is supposed to be, how exciting, and yet for you, it's no more fun than drinking a cup of tepid tea. Have you become too old for sex? Why doesn't your husband have erections any more?

These and many others are problems shared by thousands of women and many of them don't know who to turn to for advice. Your doctor may seem the obvious person but, unfortunately, as many women find out when they do summon up their courage to consult him, he is as embarrassed and uneasy talking about sex as they are. He has his problems too. He will have been taught little or nothing about psycho-sexual difficulties during his medical training. He may feel that counselling patients about sex is not part of his job. He may have sexual difficulties himself.

There are a few GPs who do take a special interest in sexual problems and have done an extra training to improve their under-standing, and if you are lucky enough to know such a doctor then he may be the best person to help you. Otherwise you would do better to contact one of the organizations mentioned on page 47. There are also some useful books to read. Particularly recommended are the following: *The Hite Report* by Shere Hite (Talmy Franklin 1977), *Our Bodies Ourselves*, edited by Angela Phillips and Jill Rakusen (Penguin 1978) and *Getting Clear: Body Work for Women* by A.K. Rush (Wildwood House 1974).

If you don't like the idea of talking to a doctor, or anyone else for that matter about your sexual problems but feel that you need treatment, then you could try doing your own sex therapy with the help of *Treat Yourself to Sex* by Paul Brown and Carolyn Faulder (Dent 1978) which is based on the work done in the sex therapy clinics run by the National Marriage Guidance Association.

Sometimes you will want to visit your doctor when you don't feel ill but you think that you need a check-up. You have heard about the need for women to have smear tests to check for cervical cancer and to have breast examinations against the possibility of breast cancer.

The *cervical smear* test should be done once a year, preferably from the age of 25 but certainly after the age of 35. For what happens when the doctor takes a smear see page 19. The specimen is sent away for examination in a laboratory to check if there are any abnormal cells.

If there are, you will have to go into hospital for a minor operation called a biopsy which involves cutting away some of the cervix. This heals quickly and does not affect your future fertility. The advantage of having a regular smear test is that if cancer cells are detected in good time, the disease can be arrested almost before it has started. However, if the test shows that the cancer is more advanced, then a total hysterectomy may be necessary.

You should examine your *breasts* once a month, preferably immediately after menstruation, but as the chances of breast cancer increase with a woman's age and the most vulnerable period is in her menopausal years between 45 and 55, it is important to continue examining your breasts throughout your life.

These are the warning signs to look out for:
any unusual lump or thickening
discharge from the nipple
alteration in the shape of the breast
any pain or discomfort
any distortion or puckering in the nipple area

Look at *The New Women's Health Handbook* for clear pictures showing you how to do a breast examination, or pick up one of the leaflets issued by the Women's National Cancer Control Campaign which are available in many clinics and doctor's waiting rooms. Another good tip for checking your breasts is to feel them all over from time to time with soapy hands in your bath.

If you do notice a change in your breasts, go to your doctor immediately. Most doctors will take you seriously, do a manual examination themselves and if they do find a lump or other abnormality send you straight off to a consultant for further tests. *Don't delay this second appointment for any reason whatever.* If there is something wrong it is vital that action be taken at once, but take comfort from the fact that only one in five women who go to their doctor with a lump turn out to have breast cancer.

There are just a few doctors around who are reluctant to examine women's breasts or pooh-pooh their anxieties. If you are unlucky enough to have a doctor like this, don't let him put you off. It is your body. You know it better than anyone else and if there is something wrong with it, you will be the first to know about it.

Explain why you are worried. If he dismisses your fears or suggests that you wait a bit to see if the condition gets any worse — this is appalling but it does happen — insist on seeing another doctor. If may cause a mildly unpleasant scene but remember, this is your right and it is your life in your hands.

13 Ill health

There are other times in your life when you know you must go to the doctor because you feel ill or you have some abnormal symptoms. Among the most common problems affecting women of all ages are vaginal infections. These show themselves fairly immediately by an *abnormal* vaginal discharge which is different in colour, substance and smell from the normal discharge you have. Often it is accompanied by a feeling of itchiness or acute soreness as well, depending on what is causing the infection. These are some of the most common infections:

Candidiasis (Thrush) caused by a yeast organism. Occasionally it is passed on sexually by a man who is not too careful about hygiene but other causes are reaction to the Pill or to antibiotics which kill off the natural vaginal bacteria which normally keep this and similar infections at bay. It's not serious but it is uncomfortable, especially if it keeps recurring.

Cystitis is inflammation of the bladder causing a need to pee every few minutes when there is no urine, an acute burning sensation and sometimes blood in the urine. About 80 per cent of women get cystitis at some time in their lives, but for some it becomes a persistent and very distressing and uncomfortable affliction which can seriously affect their life. Medical treatment is necessary but if this doesn't solve the problem look at a book called *Understanding Cystitis* by Angela Kilmartin (Pan 1975) and a leaflet called *Self-Help in Cystitis* which is available free from the U & I Club (for address see list at end of book) on receipt of a stamped addressed envelope.

Trichomoniasis (Trich) is caused by a one-celled parasite usually found in the vagina though men have it too. It's the commonest cause of vaginal discharge (usually grey-green in colour, thin and foamy) and should be treated as soon as it's detected, although many women are unaware that they have it. Very often it is sexually transmitted by men who have no symptoms.

It's very important that you get medical attention and treatment as soon as possible for these and similar conditions. Whatever you do, *don't* wash your vagina just before your visit as the doctor will need to examine you and possibly take a swab of the discharge so that it can be analysed in the laboratory.

You may find it difficult and embarrassing to talk to your GP about this kind of illness, especially if you dread him asking you searching questions about your sex life because you think he will disapprove of the answers. But the questions have to be asked and the examination must be made if the doctor is not to run the risk of overlooking something serious. Some GPs are more reluctant even than their patients to talk about these problems and they may try to take the easy way out simply by writing out a prescription without making an examination. Although you may both feel temporarily let off the hook, remember that it's your health which is at stake.

If you feel you can't communicate satisfactorily with your GP about these problems, then go to a Special Clinic which is attached to a large hospital. Here you can be sure of being treated in an anonymous way. You are given a number and the doctors who examine and treat you have no interest in you other than to cure you. Lots of questions will be asked and you must answer them all, truthfully and as completely as possible. This is especially important if there is a possibility that your illness has been caught through sexual intercourse with someone who is infected. You will then be asked to give their name(s) and address(es) so that they may be traced by a social worker. This is not betraying them. The social worker will carry out his or her enquiries as discreetly as possible and the sole purpose of giving this information is to enable your sexual contacts to be found and warned of the necessity for treatment.

Just occasionally, even in a Special Clinic where the doctors are trained not to make moral judgements, you may detect a hint of disapproval in the doctor's manner, especially if you admit to having slept with several people. Certainly you run more risk of infection if you do, but apart from pointing this out, the doctor has no business to indicate an opinion about how you conduct your sex life. Next time you need treatment, either go to a different clinic or ask for a different doctor.

In addition to the foregoing list there is a group of much more dangerous infections which are only transmitted through sexual intercourse. These are the venereal diseases of syphilis and gonorrhoea which require immediate medical treatment if they are not to threaten your health and eventually your life.

Both syphilis and gonorrhoea are particularly difficult to detect in women because they don't produce symptoms like a vaginal discharge. Both, however, can be treated successfully with penicillin, if caught early enough, so you must go to a Special Clinic immediately if you suspect that you have had sex with someone who is infected.

For a clear, diagrammatic description of a number of other minor and more serious disorders, including syphilis and gonorrhoea look at *Woman's Body, An Owner's Manual* by the Diagram Group (Paddington Press 1977). *The New Women's Health Handbook* edited by Nancy MacKeith is also very helpful, particularly about the side-effects of using certain drugs.

14 Why it helps to talk to other women

All through this handbook we have been referring to the relationship between a doctor and his women patients. For each to learn how to talk to the other is very important if women are to get all the help, advice and treatment that they need to keep themselves in a state of good health. However, there is another way in which women can help themselves and that is by talking and listening to one another.

Up to a point this is what they have always done, and what a lot of jokes at their expense there have been about old wives' tales. women's gossip, etc! Much of what mothers tell their daughters and friends tell each other is the only information women ever get about themselves and their bodies, so if it is inaccurate or misleading or alarmist it undoubtedly does more harm than good.

However, just as often hearing about other women's experiences can be valuable, enriching and enlightening. It can be a source of support and a springboard for action. Talking about your own experience to a sympathetic woman may help you put your own problem into perspective or help her to understand the one which is bothering her.

Until recently, women did as they were told in matters concerning their health, convinced that doctor knew best. Today we have a more healthily sceptical frame of mind and some of the most important reforms in health care are being led by women's groups. (For a comprehensive list look at *The Women's Directory*). The new women's movement has also had an important influence on the way we think about ourselves — not as wombs on legs as one doctor with an amazing lack of taste once said to me — but as total human beings with the same right to self-fulfilment as men. Today, women are writing and talking to each other as never before. It's worth listening to what they have to say.

ADDRESSES

Family Planning Clinics are listed in your local telephone directory under 'Family Planning'.

Brook Advisory Centres Headquarters are in London at 233 Tottenham Court Road, WC1. Tel: 01-323 1522 and clinics all over the country. (Addresses in your local telephone directory).

British Pregnancy Advisory Service, Headquarters are in Birmingham at 1st Floor, Guildhall Buildings, Navigation Street, Birmingham B2 4BT. Tel: 021-643 1461. Branches in London, Brighton, Leeds, Manchester, Liverpool and other large city centres.

Pregnancy Advisory Service, 40 Margaret Street, London W.1. Tel: 01-409 0281.

National Marriage Guidance Council. Headquarters at Little Church Street, Rugby. Tel: Rugby 73241 and branches all over the country. (Addresses in your local telephone directory).

The Association of Sexual and Marital Therapists, 79 Harley Street, London, W.1. For a complete list of all the centres where treatment for sexual problems is available and names of individual local therapists who either you or your doctor can contact, write to the above address enclosing a large stamped addressed envelope.

BUPA Medical Centre Ltd, Webb House, 210 Pentonville Road, London N.1. Tel: 01-278 4565.

Marie Stopes House, The Well-Woman Centre, 108 Whitfield Street, London W.1. Tel: 01-388 0662.

Women's Health Care, 16 Seymour Street, London W.1. Tel: 01-486 4069. Will provide you with a list of hospitals with menopausal clinics and doctors specializing in menopausal problems.

Health Education Council, 78 New Oxford Street, W.C.1. Tel: 01-637 1881. Produce pamphlets on most aspects of health: information and advisory service.

U & I Club, 22 Gerrard Road, London, N.1.